How To Be STRONG And FAST After 60

Seniors' Guide to Strength Training for Better Balance, Mobility, and Everyday Living

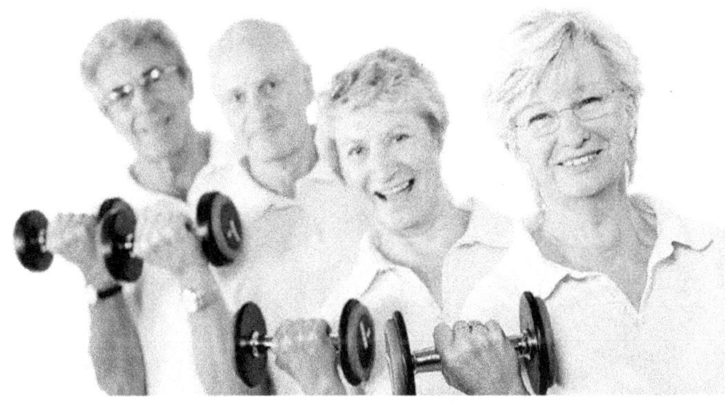

Dr. Cindy Dye

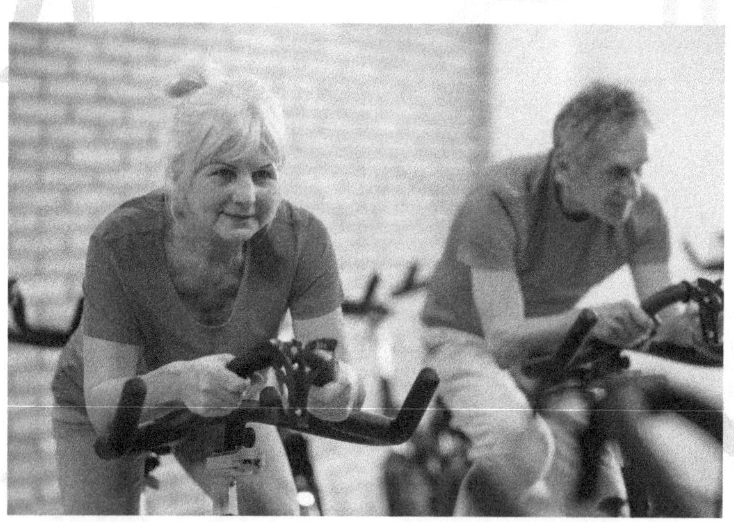

TABLE OF CONTENTS

TABLE OF CONTENTS 3

INTRODUCTION 6

A Quick Reminder 8

Advantages of Strength Training 9

THE BASIC STRENGTH TRAINING FORMULA 16

STRENGTH TRAINING RULES 19

The Best Recommended Weights For Seniors 29

NUTRITION: EATING TO GET YOU HEALTHY & STRONG 30

RECOMMENDED RECIPES FOR THE WORKOUT 38

.... 48

EXERCISE FOR PEOPLE WITH RESTRICTIVE LIFESTYLE 50

Exercise Programs for Restrictive Lifestyles 50

The Time-Crunched 50

The Desk Dweller 51

The Travel Warrior 52

The Homebody 53

EXERCISE FOR PEOPLE WITH SEDENTARY TO MODERATE ACTIVE LIFESTYLE 55

Couch Potato to Mover 55

Moderately Active to Fitness Enthusiast 56

Pro-Tips for Both Levels 57

Exercise for People with Active and Able Lifestyle 58

4 WEEKS EXERCISE CHALLENGE 62

Sedentary to Mover 62

Moderately Active to Fitness Enthusiast....................................63

Conclusion...65

Frequent Asks Questions........................68

Exercise Log Book..................................72

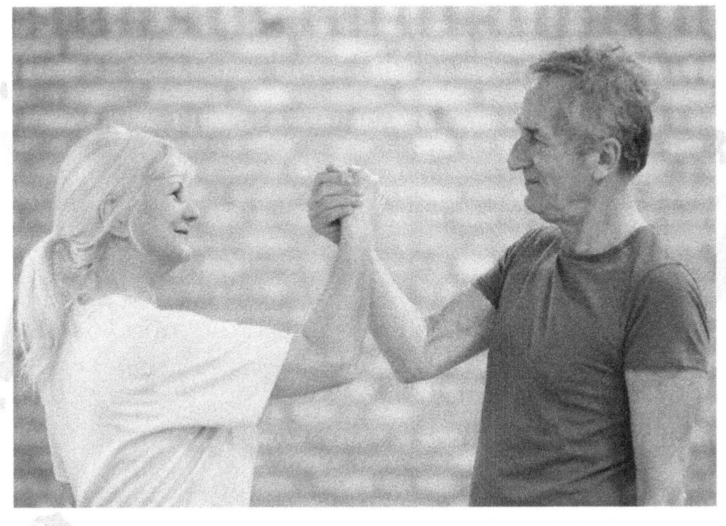

INTRODUCTION

Life is much easier!

Remember chasing fireflies as a kid, legs pumping, laughter echoing on the summer breeze? Or dominating the high school soccer field, the wind whipping past your face as you scored the winning goal? Where did that raw power, that exhilarating speed, go? Is it forever locked away in the dusty halls of youth?

Not a chance.

I wasn't always the silver-haired dynamo you see on the cover. At 58, I was on the fast track to becoming a statistic - hunched over, shuffling along, resigned to the ache in my knees and the creak in my back. My doctor's words still sting: "It's all downhill from here, Margaret."

Downhill? I wasn't buying it. My spirit still thrummed with the memory of movement, the forgotten thrill of pushing my limits. And so, I decided to fight back. Not just against wrinkles and grey hairs, but against the insidious notion that age equals decline.

This book is the chronicle of my rebellion. It's a road map, a battle cry, an invitation to every restless soul trapped in a slowing body. Forget what you've ever learned about aging. Forget the limitations society whispers in your ear.

I'm here to tell you, with every ache-defying sprint, every heart-pounding climb, that strength and speed are not exclusive to youth. They're embers waiting to be rekindled, even after 60.

"How to Be Strong and Fast After 60" isn't a magic potion. It's a blueprint, a set of tools forged in the fire of my own personal transformation. You'll find no fad diets or miracle cures, just science-backed strategies, practical exercises, and a whole lot of tough love.

We'll delve into the secrets of building muscle and boosting metabolism, even if your AARP card arrives in the mail every month. We'll conquer joint pain, master balance, and rediscover the joy of a body that moves with purpose.

This book isn't just about running marathons (though, why not?). It's about reclaiming your life, one step, one push-up, one burst of laughter at your own reflection in the mirror at a time. It's about proving that 60 is not the end, but the beginning of a whole new adventure.

Ready to turn back the clock on your body and reignite your inner athlete? Turn the page. Your revolution starts now.

A Quick Reminder

If you this boo, I'd really appreciate it if you leave a review on Amazon.

Review really help independent writers like myself get in front of the right audience and help more people

Thank you so much in advance.

Loss of muscular mass and power to achieve the things you want and need to do, IS AVOIDABLE!

AND .... If you have already realized you have lost strength and muscle....

It is REVERSIBLE as well!

Advantages of Strength Training

Younger, Stronger & More Efficient Muscles

Loss of strength and muscular mass is a natural part of aging.

Sarcopenia is the age-related weakening and atrophy of the muscles.

Sarcopenia may have several causes.The good news is that reduced physical activity over time is the sole cause of sarcopenia in most people.

Sarcopenia is **NOT** only a natural part of becoming older.

As a result of being unused, it is certain to happen.

Muscle cells shrink and weaken when our level of physical activity decreases.

By doing **MORE** physical activity, and practicing strength exercises, you may reverse the effects of sarcopenia, essentially reversing the aging process of your muscles and enhancing their effectiveness.

Look Better - Lose Weight & Improve Posture

We **ALL** want to appear better!

I'm sure it's fair to state that all of us, both men and women, regardless of age, appear better with a good amount of muscle on our frames.

We also appear healthy with proper posture.

With constant strength exercise (along with a healthy diet) you will increase muscle mass, improve your posture (by resolving muscular imbalances), and decrease body fat.

When you build muscle mass and reduce fat, you get what's usually referred to as that "toned" look, which I know many of you reading this are pursuing.

Cardiovascular exercise (jogging, running, riding a bike, boxing, skipping, and so on) is the sort of activity widely regarded to be optimal for fat reduction.

However, I'd go as far as to argue that appropriate strength training may do just as much, if not more, for weight loss and weight management than cardiovascular exercise does.

Research reveals that strength training leads in reductions of abdominal fat in both older men and women.

And subsequent study reveals, completing strength training resulted in just one-third as much fat growth over two years compared to those not doing strength training. Demonstrating the impact of strength training on managing weight.

Now I am not advocating to quit practicing cardiovascular exercise, particularly if you love it.

There are advantages in conducting cardiovascular exercise for everyone over 60. However, if you don't want to, you may become healthy, strong and look your best by performing solely correct strength training.

"Exercise is king. Nutrition is queen. Put them together and you've got a kingdom."

Jack Lalanne

Improve Physical & Mental Health & Get More, Quality Sleep

Along with being stronger, developing muscle, shedding weight and improving posture, strength training can improve physical and mental health.

For improvements in our physical health, strength training may lower the risk factors of metabolic syndrome, decreasing blood pressure and reducing the risk of cardiovascular disease.

It has beneficial effects on cholesterol levels and body fat percentage.

Strength training may have a role in improving insulin resistance associated with aging and prevent the development of diabetes.

Strength training may also contribute to many mental health advantages.

After constant strength training, you will feel improved confidence, self-esteem and have more vitality. And, it is a powerful strategy for decreasing stress and reducing anxiety, depression and fatigue.

Moreover, if you want to maintain your memory in top form strength exercise may enhance numerous elements of cognition, memory and memory-related tasks in healthy older persons.

And we all know the health advantages of having a good night's sleep. Resistance exercise can improve sleep quality and quantity.

Decrease Joint & Other Pain. Strengthen & Avoid Brittle Bones (Help With Arthritis & Osteoporosis)

Strength training can prevent and minimize discomfort. Studies have shown improvement in pain in persons who have fibromyalgia, lower back pain and arthritis.

With painful joints illnesses such as arthritis, by strengthening the muscles, ligaments and tendons around an afflicted joint, we may minimize the stress exerted on the joint, decreasing pain sensations.

Strength exercise may also be effective to prevent, and reverse osteoporosis. Studies have revealed increases in bone mineral density, helping to prevent and strengthen brittle bones.

Furthermore, stronger persons are predisposed to have greater bone mineral density compared to those who are weaker.

Increased strength and muscle mass can decrease one's risk of falls when paired with increased bone mineral density, dramatically lowers the risk of fractures and other injuries due to falls.

Strength training has also been proven to be beneficial in improving balance and correcting age-related changes in gait speed (how quickly you walk), stride length (the size of your step), cadence (the pace of your walk) and toe clearance (cleaning your toes off the floor with each step) . All variables that are damaged, may put one at danger of falling.

As you can see, there are many, many long term advantages of strength training and I hope by now I've got you over the line to begin strength training and start improving your life, and health.

Certainly, to enjoy all the advantages and practice strength training properly, it is necessary you do strength training appropriately by following a few procedures which we will go over in the next part.

> *"Age is no barrier. It's a limitation you put on your mind."* - **Jackie Joyner-Kersee**

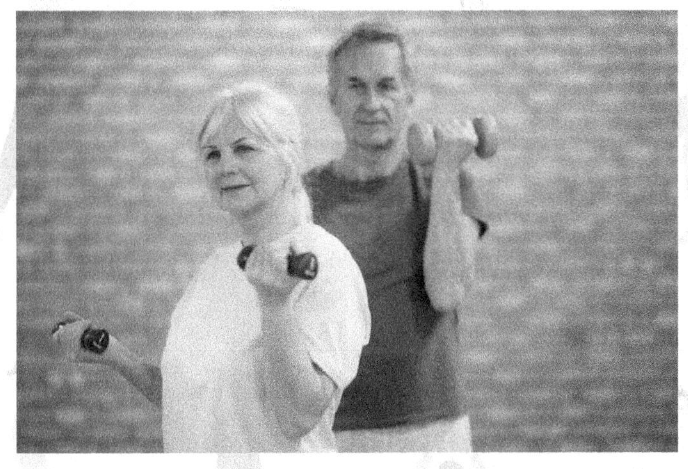

THE BASIC STRENGTH TRAINING FORMULA

THE BASIC FORMULA FOR STRENGTH

LIFT HEAVY THINGS + STAY CONSISTENT & PROGRESS THE EXERCISE + EAT PROPER NUTRITION = STRONG MUSCLES + EASIER LIFE

1. Do exercise involving resistance in some way, whether body weight exercises or utilizing equipment (E.G. Weights or resistance bands).

Make sure your muscles are being worked hard enough throughout each exercise (they grow weary - not exhausted), within a certain set and repetition range (explained in a section to follow).

2. Do this consistently each week, being careful to progress the workouts when it gets too easy. Continue to challenge yourself.

You may accomplish this by increasing the repetition range (if performing body weight exercises), practicing a more demanding variant of the exercise, lowering rest time, or by raising the weight/resistance.

3. Support your strength exercise with proper diet. Do not overlook the significance of appropriate diet for building strength and muscular growth. To lose weight, getting your food properly is up to 80-90% of the issue. If you're under-eating or have a bad diet, your strength increases will be substantially limited. (Nutrition for strength will also be mentioned below).

Do these three steps, and you **WILL** grow stronger.

It really I.S. this easy! You don't need to make it much more difficult than this!

There are a few extra nuances we'll go over to ensure you perform each step perfectly, but this is the foundation of it.

Stick to this formula, and you cannot go wrong!

Now, let's get into the nitty-gritty of strength training, beginning with basic principles to guarantee you get the most out of it and most importantly, do it safely.

> *"There's more to life than training, but training is what puts more in your life."* - **Brooks Kubik**

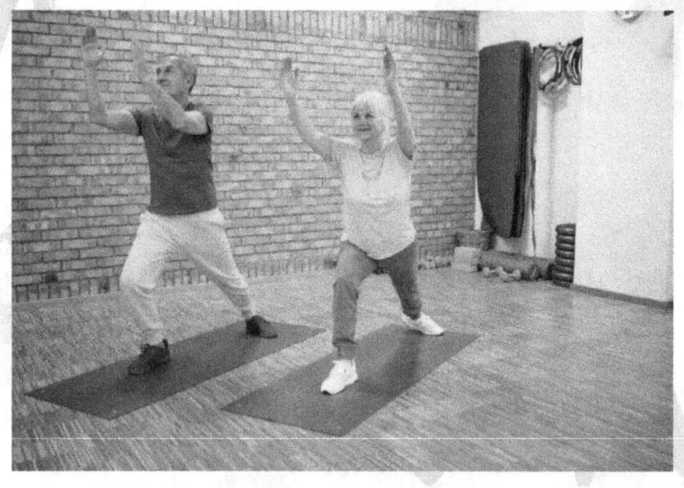

STRENGTH TRAINING RULES

So, now we know the fundamental, no-fail formula necessary to grow stronger and gain muscle, and it's nearly time we get into the real strength training.

However, before we delve right into it, we must go over some fundamental strength training regulations, which when attended to, will keep you safe throughout and assist you to get the most out of your strength training.

RULE 1: SEE YOUR DOCTOR

I'm sure you know the drill....

As with any workout, there are hazards involved, and you want to make sure you can practice strength training without putting yourself at risk.

To give yourself (and me) piece of mind, consult your Doctor!

Get the all-clear before you begin strength training.

Also consulting a Health Professional, such as a Physiotherapist may be a good idea before you start strength training for the first time.

By doing this, you may learn to execute the exercises with assistance and any areas of weakness can be handled with first.

Once you've done the following, and you're all ready to go, you may safely begin your exercise.

RULE 2: ALWAYS DO A WARM-UP!

First and foremost, before commencing any activity, always and I mean ALWAYS complete a warm-up!

A warm-up is incredibly crucial, particularly with strength exercise and even more so as we become older.

Properly warming-up before working out is vital to prepare your body for what follows.

By practicing at least a 5-minute warm-up before your real program, will not only lower your chances of being hurt, or other difficulties, but you also prepare your body ready for the strength workouts that follow.

The warm-up supports you by waking up your muscles (and yourself), lubricating your joints, and enhancing your range of motion, enabling you to get more out of the exercise.

To make things simpler for you, I have designed two warm-up routines which are easy to follow.

RULES 3: LEARN FIRST & USE GOOD EXERCISE TECHNIQUE

With each new exercise, mastering the right exercise technique first, before increasing the weight, is a requirement!

If new to exercising, I suggest beginning with body weight exercises and reserve resistance bands and lifting weights for later, when you have acquired the technique and become a bit stronger.

This will guarantee no harm and help you get the most out of the workouts, making them more effective.

To make sure that you're appropriately completing the exercises, obtain a professional evaluation, work with a training partner or execute the exercises in front of a mirror so you can see how it appears.

This manner, you can always monitor your workout technique and adjust it if it begins to deteriorate.

Once you become comfortable with your technique and feel that body weight isn't pushing you enough longer, it is time to bring in some resistance bands or weights.

Only until you have perfect workout technique should you consider about bringing in extra weight/resistance to the exercises.

Good exercise technique is going to accomplish much more in obtaining you the outcomes you are looking than the quantity of weight you are exercising with. So keep patient!

Once you start making progress, the idea is to improve your strength gradually, and this can only be done safely, by gradually raising the weight.

Your body will appreciate you, you'll remain injury-free, and you'll make fantastic progress over time!

RULE 4: ALWAYS EASE INTO EXERCISE

When commencing strength training with weights (or bands) for the first time, get started by lifting lighter, and performing less than you're capable of (fewer repetitions and sets).

This will get your body acclimated to the workout **AND** enable you to prevent any soreness or damage.

Soreness **(DOMS)** the following days after strength exercise is perfectly normal and to be anticipated. But, you don't want to be in a whole world of agony, which might happen if you do too much!

Once you've mastered the strength exercises and got your body adapted to them, after a few weeks, you may then begin doing more and more.

Another error I regularly see, is individuals quit performing exercise, or physical activity, for a long period (for different reasons) and finally when they get back into the exercise, they attempt to start back up where they left off. Avoid doing this!

You need to take a few steps back before you get to where you were. This will lessen any risks of becoming hurt and boost your outcomes in the long term.

Always ease into action, whatever it is, particularly weights.

By doing this, you'll avoid any complications and be back to where you were in no time!

RULE 5: DON'T LIFT TO HEAVY

There may come a point when you are tempted to raise bigger weights than you are capable of.

You constantly want to be pushing yourself, but you don't ever want to be going beyond your limitations, leaving correct workout technique behind and putting yourself at danger of injury.

Heavier weights with poor workout technique accomplishes nothing to grow your muscles stronger and puts additional pressure on other regions of your body.

Keep your weights within your ability and **SLOWLY** raise the weight over time.

RULE 6: DON'T OVERDO IT, GIVE ADEQUATE REST & NEVER PUSH INTO PAIN

This one is fairly similar to what we spoke about earlier - employing a weight that's too heavy for you.

But pushing oneself over the boundaries doesn't necessary imply utilizing too much weight; it may relate to over-exercising too.

Getting stronger does not need lengthy, strenuous workout sessions. This is unneeded, placing enormous levels of stress on your body, and it will work against you in attaining the results you desire.

You also want to give yourself recuperation between strength training. When we use our muscles with resistance, our muscular tissue breaks down. Our body understands it needs to adapt to the additional pressures it is under and will begin healing and grow stronger, bigger muscles to be able to withstand these workouts again.

Our body restores itself via relaxation, sleep and good diet. So always allow yourself ample recuperation between strength training sessions, particularly in the beginning.

I suggest a day in between each strength training and remember to eat properly and always obtaining a good night's sleep.

Finally, remember, workouts should **NEVER** cause you any discomfort. You could have a stretching sensation, weariness or that burning kind sense of your muscles being pushed, and pain the following day. But you should never experience pain.

This is why it's crucial to listen to your body and quit if it's giving you discomfort. You will know when it doesn't seem right!

Also stop if you develop any other unexpected symptoms, such as chest discomfort, dizziness, or feeling faint.

RULE 7: STICK TO THE CORRECT SETS AND REP RANGES

To get the most out of your strength training, keep to the right repetition and set ranges.

We'll explore this in a future part, but for now, know there is a quantity of the workout we should keep to, which will assist us develop stronger. And we'll grow stronger quicker.

RULE 8: STAY CONSISTENT, ALWAYS BE CHALLENGING YOURSELF & PROGRESS THE EXERCISES

The last tip to follow to guarantee you build your strength is to be consistent.

Doing a strength training every now and then is not going to increase your strength.

You have to be performing strength training, without fail, each week. (We'll consider the frequency of workouts next).

Along with this consistency, as you grow stronger, you also want to be pushing your muscles by raising the repetition ranges (if performing body weight exercises) or raise the amount of weight (or the resistance of the bands), or you must practice more demanding activities.

If you don't continue to push yourself, your strength will ultimately plateau out and you won't become any stronger.

Always be pushing yourself! And remain constant!

Follow these tips for your strength training to practice strength training safely and to truly achieve benefits.

With a clearer sense of what to accomplish, we now get to the strength training factors that will best develop your strength – beginning with how many times to exercise each week.

> *"Exercise not only changes your body, it changes your mind, your attitude and your mood."* - **Gene Tunney**

The Best Recommended Weights For Seniors

For weights, I also advocate acquiring a modest set to save money and to allow for advancement as your strength grows.

For beginners, I advise beginning with 1-5kg (2-11lbs) weights They are an excellent starting weight which will help you to master the movements, and they provide opportunity for improvement.

When you outgrow these weights (a nice issue to have), you may look at getting larger weights.

Additionally, for those who have a strong degree of strength, you may need to start with bigger weights.

If you continue with the same modest weights, your body will not become any stronger.

Progress the weight, by lifting heavier, and your body will adapt and grow stronger.

If you travel to your local department shop, you can simply pick up a set of dumbbells.

NUTRITION: EATING TO GET YOU HEALTHY & STRONG

Eating healthily is critical for health and well-being, and is also necessary for growing muscle and enhancing strength. **AND** reducing the waistline.

To grow stronger and develop muscle efficiently, we need to be ingesting enough calories/energy from excellent quality protein, fat and carbohydrate sources.

We also need to consume appropriate micronutrients (vitamins and minerals) to support our body's biological functions and maintain ourselves healthy.

When we are taking in too few calories, or consuming mainly junk foods, we don't receive in all our essential nutrients, resulting to worse health and loss of muscle and strength.

Nutrition is a big subject, difficult to discuss in this tutorial. I could create a whole new guide on it. I'll reserve it for a later date, however.

For now, optimize your diet by trying your best to avoid junk meals, and start receiving the ideal number of calories from nutrient-rich foods.

There are specific nutrients you want to be receiving enough levels of to aid enhance your strength (and health) likewise. That being protein, vitamin D, magnesium and calcium, since low-level consumption of these nutrients has been associated to lower strength, muscular mass and physical performance in seniors.

Let's take a long look these nutrients:

PROTEIN

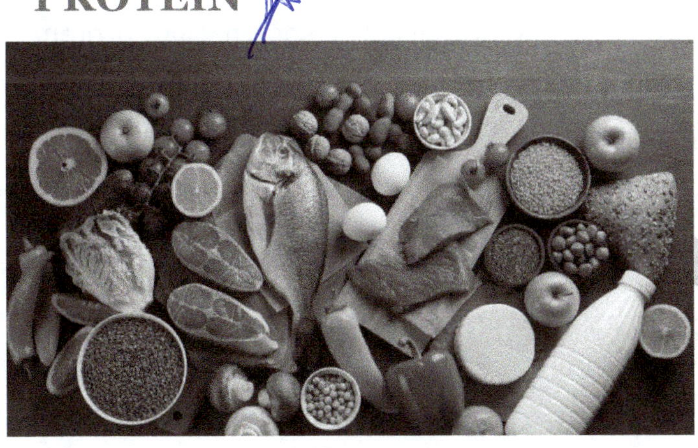

Protein is crucial for preserving muscular mass, and strength, as one grows older, and it's fairly typical not to be receiving enough.

The Australian Dietary Guidelines recommend that 15-25% of our total calorie consumption should come from protein, with a daily intake of the following:

- The RDI of protein for women aged 19–70 years is 46 grams per day.
- The RDI of protein for males aged 19-70 years is 64 grams per day.
- Women over 70 should have at least 57g per day.
- Men over 70 should have above 81g per day.

However, new studies has shown that protein consumption greater than this may be necessary to assist retain muscular strength and function into later age.

The European Society for Clinical Nutrition and Metabolism (ESPEN) gives the following guidelines, based on studies gathered:

1. For healthy seniors - at least 1.0 to 1.2 g protein/kg body weight/day is suggested.

2. For seniors who are at risk of malnutrition because they have an acute or chronic disease, the diet should offer 1.2 to 1.5 g protein/kg body weight/day.

3. For seniors with serious sickness or injury - even greater intake of 1.2 to 1.5 g protein/kg body weight/day may be recommended.

ESPEN also advised regular exercise and resistance training to preserve health and muscular strength and function.

To discover more about protein and receive suggestions on how to obtain more protein in your diet, click here.

VITAMIN D

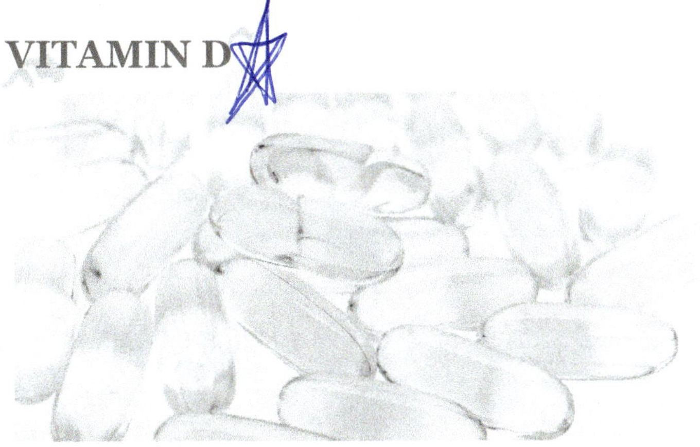

We create vitamin D when our skin is exposed to the sun. As we become older, we tend to spend less time in the sun, particularly in the winter months, making vitamin D shortages more frequent.

Vitamin D is needed in older age for bone strength, muscular function, and to avoid falls.

Low vitamin D levels are connected with reduced muscle mass and poor athletic performance.

Aim to obtain 20 minutes' direct sunshine everyday, avoiding the warmest period of the day. This keeps your vitamin D levels topped up, helping you stay healthy and powerful. Make cautious not to overuse it and burn your skin.

MAGNESIUM

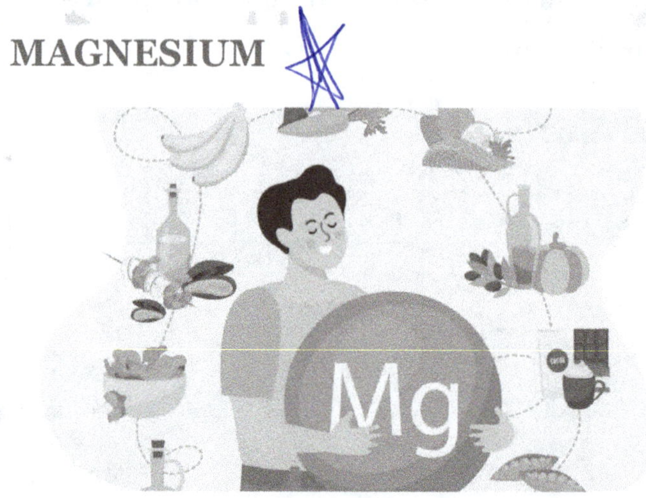

Magnesium is another mineral we need for optimum health.

Magnesium is necessary for many of our body's basic activities, including producing energy, for neuron and muscle function, manufacturing DNA, bone and protein, and for a healthy heart and robust immune system.

Decreased magnesium intakes have been shown in seniors who have poorer muscular mass and strength.

Furthermore, intake of magnesium has been linked to increased physical function and strength in seniors.

I'll be producing an article shortly to assist you learn more about magnesium and receive suggestions on how to acquire extra magnesium in your diet. (keep tuned for this).

> *"Diet is the essential key to all successful healing. Without a properly balanced diet, the effectiveness of herbal treatment is very limited."* – **Michael Tierra**

CALCIUM

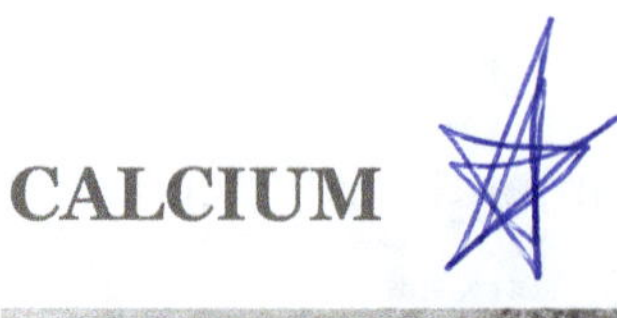

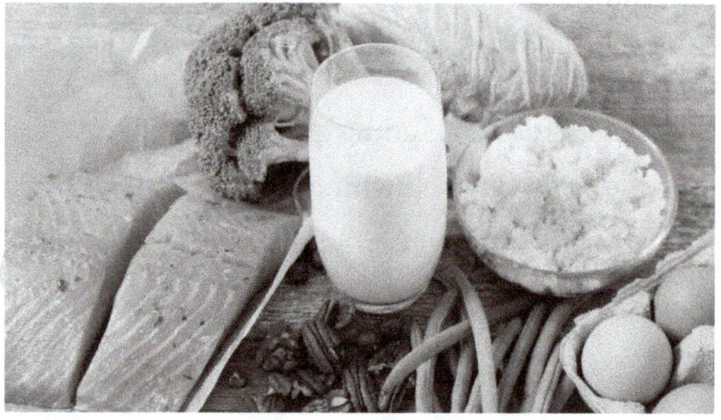

Calcium is needed for strong bones and healthy teeth. It also plays a critical part in other biological systems, such as our neurological system and the appropriate functioning of our muscles.

Our typical weight is made up of roughly two per cent calcium. This calcium is largely located in our bones and teeth – the remainder kept in our blood and tissues.

poor calcium consumption has been associated to osteoporosis, a poor bone density disorder most typically found in post-menopausal women.

Research has indicated that seniors with low calcium levels, had 3-4 times greater risk of sarcopenia and slower gait speed, compared to those with a higher calcium level

To read more about calcium and receive tips on how to acquire extra calcium in your diet.

Strength training mixed with a good diet, with appropriate calories, macronutrients (particularly protein) and micronutrients (including vitamin D, magnesium and calcium), is a solid approach of preventing sarcopenia, and living a strong and healthy life.

> *"If you eat healthily you'll feel better, have more energy, and ultimately live longer."*
>
> **- Ralph Marston**

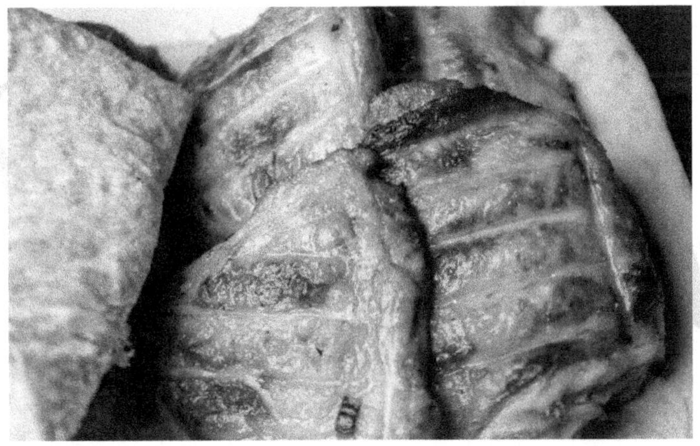

RECOMMENDED RECIPES FOR THE WORKOUT

Pre-Workout Protein Smoothie

⏰ **10 Mininues**

INGREDIENTS

1 scoop vanilla protein powder

1 cup berries

1 banana

1 cup unsweetened almond milk

½ cup spinach

¼ teaspoon cinnamon.

DIRECTIONS

1. Blend all ingredients until smooth.
2. Enjoy 30-60 minutes before your workout.

This recipes Provides sustainable energy and muscle repair.

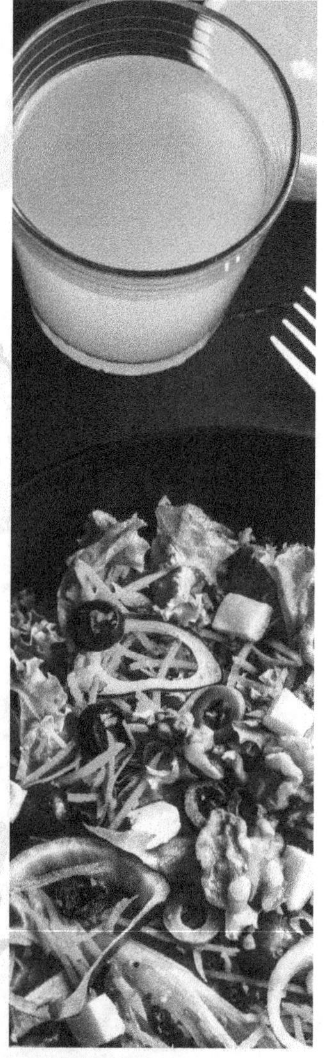

Post-Workout Recovery Oatmeal

⏰ **15 Mininues**

INGREDIENTS

½ cup rolled oats

1 cup unsweetened almond milk

1 scoop chocolate protein powder

¼ cup blueberries

1 tablespoon chopped nuts

honey to taste.

DIRECTIONS

1. Cook oats in almond milk.
2. Stir in protein powder, top with berries, nuts, and drizzle with honey.

This Recipes Replenishes carbohydrates and aids muscle recovery

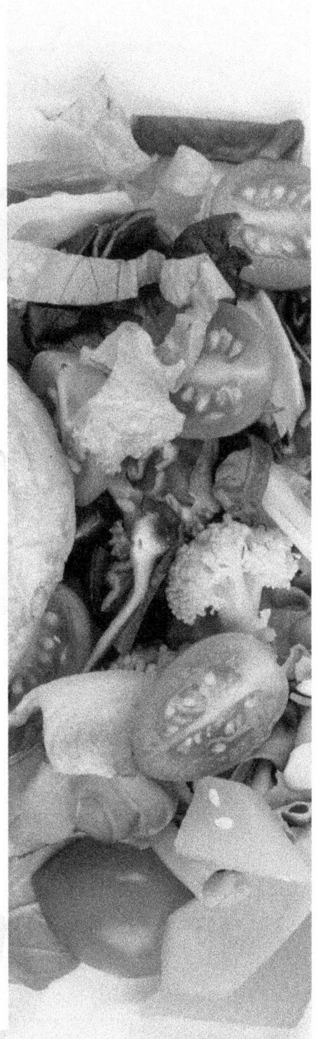

Greek Yogurt Power Parfait

5 Mininues

INGREDIENTS

1 scoop vanilla protein powder

1 cup berries

1 banana

1 cup unsweetened almond milk

½ cup spinach

¼ teaspoon cinnamon.

DIRECTIONS

3. Blend all ingredients until smooth.
4. Enjoy 30-60 minutes before your workout.

This recipes is rich in protein and calcium for muscle building and bone health.

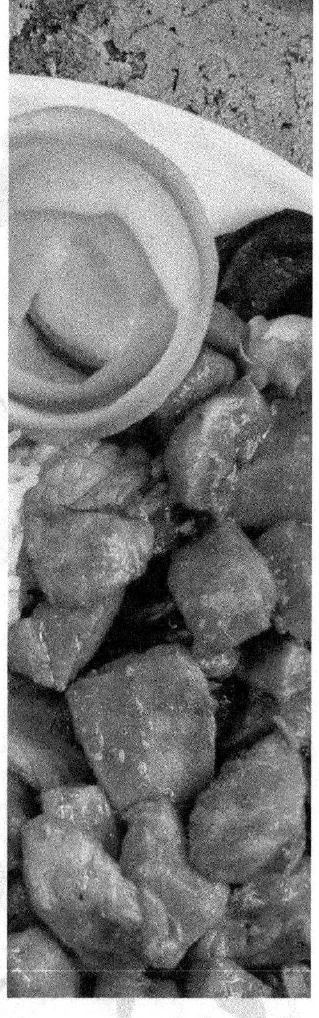

Salmon with Roasted Vegetables

⏰ **30 Mininues**

INGREDIENTS

4 salmon fillets

1 tablespoon olive oil

Salt

Pepper assorted vegetables

(broccoli, carrots, asparagus).

DIRECTIONS

1. Preheat oven to 400°F.
2. Toss vegetables with olive oil, salt, and pepper.
3. Spread on a baking sheet and roast for 15 minutes.
4. Season salmon with salt and pepper, bake for 10-12 minutes alongside vegetables.

Excellent source of lean protein and omega-3 fatty

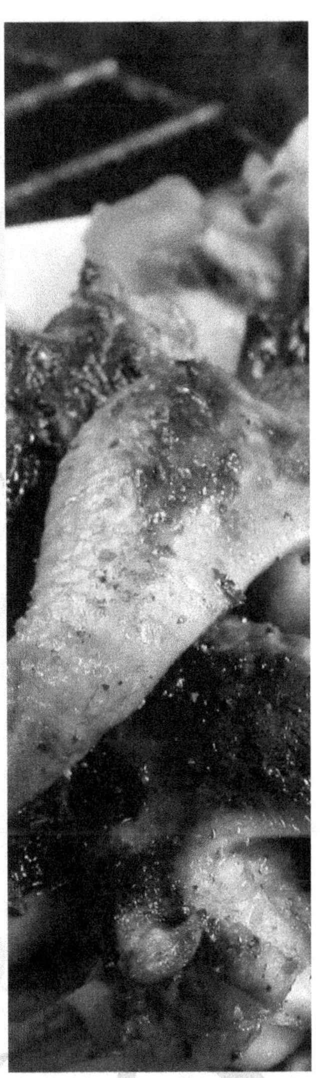

Chicken Quinoa Salad

⏰ **20 Mininues**

INGREDIENTS

1 cup cooked quinoa

1 grilled chicken breast, chopped

½ cup chopped cucumber

¼ cup crumbled feta cheese

2 tablespoons olive oil

lemon juice

Salt and pepper.

DIRECTIONS

1. Combine quinoa, chicken, cucumber, and feta cheese.
2. Whisk olive oil, lemon juice, salt, and pepper into a dressing.
3. Toss salad with dressing and enjoy.

Provides balanced carbohydrates, protein, and fiber for sustained energy.

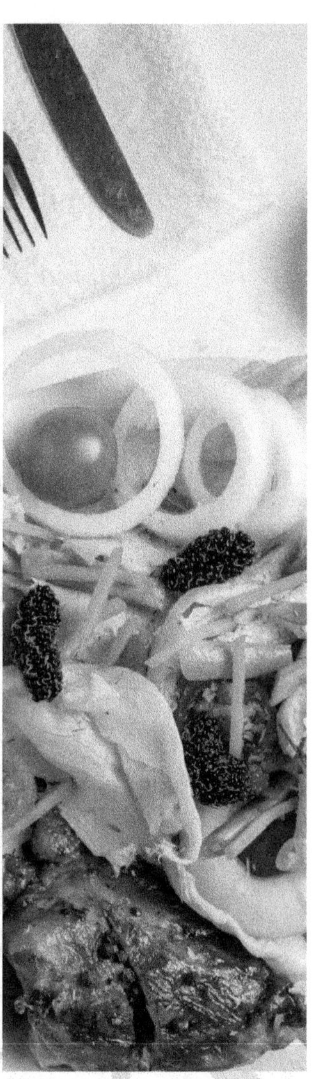

Lentil Soup with Whole Wheat Bread

⏰ **30 Mininues**

INGREDIENTS

1 cup brown lentils, 4 cups vegetable broth

1 chopped onion, 1 chopped carrot

1 chopped celery stalk, 1 clove garlic, minced

1 teaspoon dried thyme

salt, pepper, 2 slices whole wheat bread.

DIRECTIONS

1. Sauté onion, carrot, celery, and garlic in a pot.
2. Add lentils, broth, thyme, salt, and pepper.
3. Bring to a boil, then simmer for 20 minutes or until lentils are tender.
4. Serve with toasted whole wheat bread.

Packed with plant-based protein and fiber for gut health and satiety.

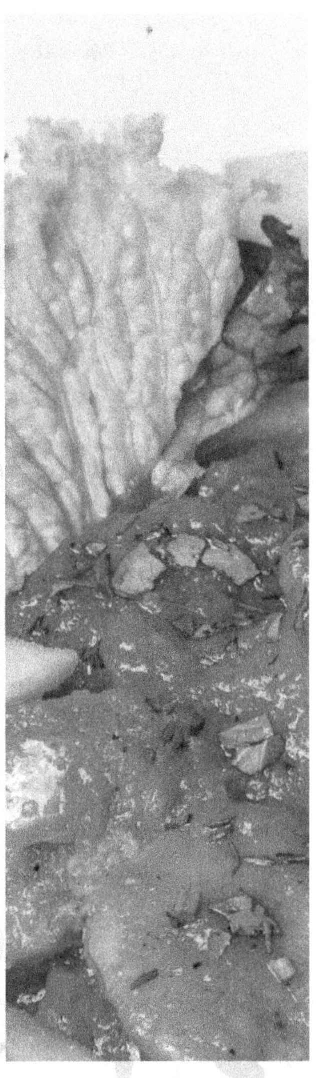

Tuna Salad Lettuce Wraps

⏰ **15 Mininues**

INGREDIENTS

2 cans tuna packed in water, drained

1 chopped avocado

¼ cup chopped celery

2 tablespoons Greek yogurt

1 tablespoon lemon juice, dill,

salt, pepper, lettuce leaves.

DIRECTIONS

1. Combine tuna, avocado, celery, yogurt, lemon juice, dill, salt, and pepper.
2. Fill lettuce leaves with tuna salad mixture and enjoy.

Light and refreshing option with healthy fats from avocado.

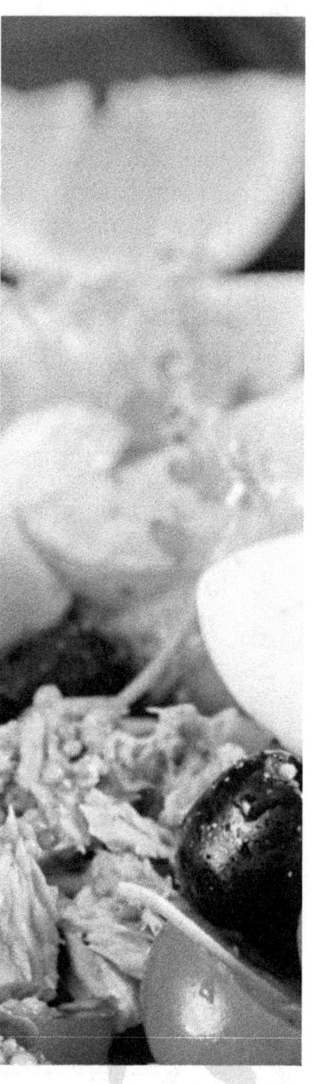

Veggie Frittata

⏰ **25 Mininues**

INGREDIENTS

6 eggs, beaten

½ cup chopped zucchini

½ cup chopped bell peppers

¼ cup chopped onion

1 tablespoon olive oil

¼ cup crumbled feta cheese

Salt and pepper.

DIRECTIONS

1. Preheat oven to 400°F.
2. Heat olive oil in an oven-safe skillet.
3. Sauté vegetables until softened.
4. Pour in eggs and top with feta cheese.
5. Bake for 15-20 minutes or until eggs are set.

Versatile and packed with vitamins and minerals from vegetables.

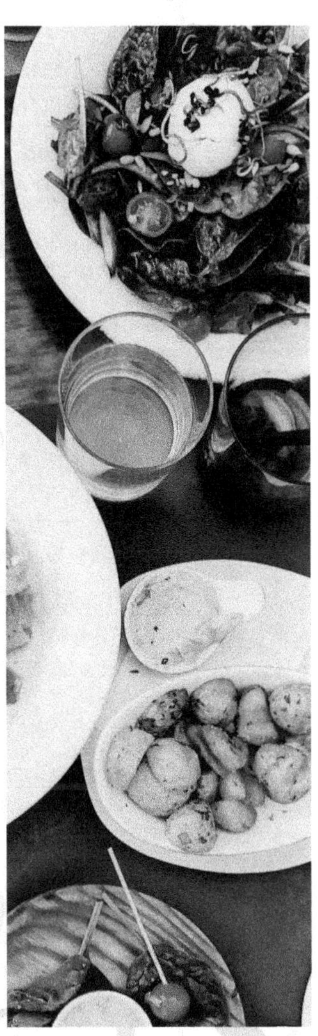

Turkey Cranberry Meatballs

20 Mininues

INGREDIENTS

1 pound ground turkey, ½ cup chopped onion

¼ cup chopped celery, ¼ cup dried cranberries

¼ cup panko breadcrumbs, 1 egg, beaten

1 tablespoon olive oil

cranberry sauce for dipping (optional).

DIRECTIONS

1. Preheat oven to 400°F.
2. Combine turkey, onion, celery, cranberries, breadcrumbs, and egg in a bowl.
3. Mix well and form into meatballs.
4. Place on a baking sheet and bake for 15-20 minutes or until cooked through.
5. Serve with cranberry sauce for dipping, if desired.

Light and refreshing option with healthy fats from avocado.

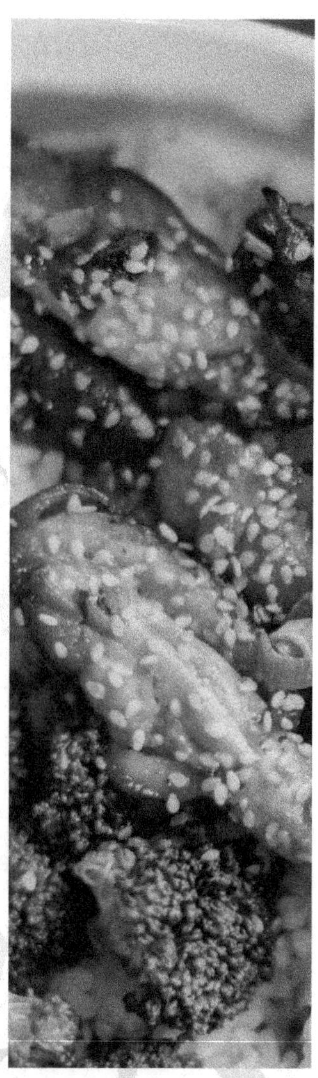

Banana Chia Pudding

Overnight

INGREDIENTS

2 mashed bananas

½ cup chia seeds

1 cup unsweetened almond milk

1 teaspoon honey

¼ teaspoon cinnamon, granola and berries for topping (optional).

DIRECTIONS

1. In a jar or container, combine mashed bananas, chia seeds, almond milk, honey, and cinnamon.
2. Stir well and refrigerate overnight.
3. Top with granola and berries before serving.

Versatile and packed with vitamins and minerals from vegetables.

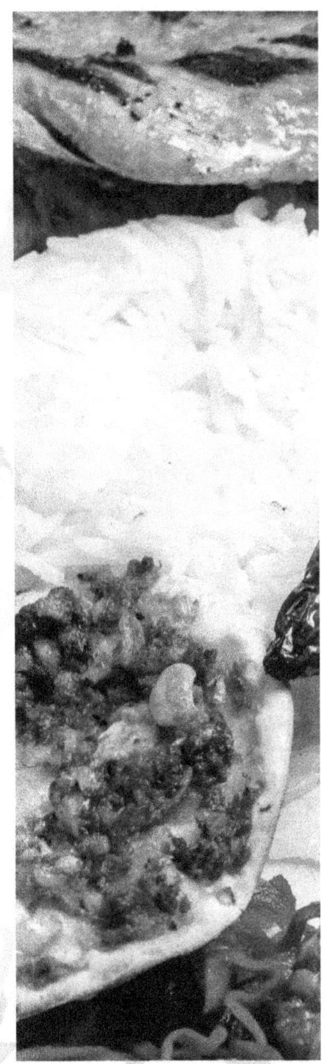

Coconut Chia Pudding with Mango and Granola

⏰ **10 Mininues**

INGREDIENTS

1/2 cup chia seeds

1 cup unsweetened coconut milk

1/4 cup sliced mango

1 tablespoon honey (optional)

1/4 cup granola

DIRECTIONS

1. In a jar or container, combine chia seeds and coconut milk.
2. Stir in honey, if using.
3. Cover and refrigerate overnight.
4. In the morning, top with sliced mango and granola.

A refreshing and portable breakfast or snack with healthy fats and fiber.

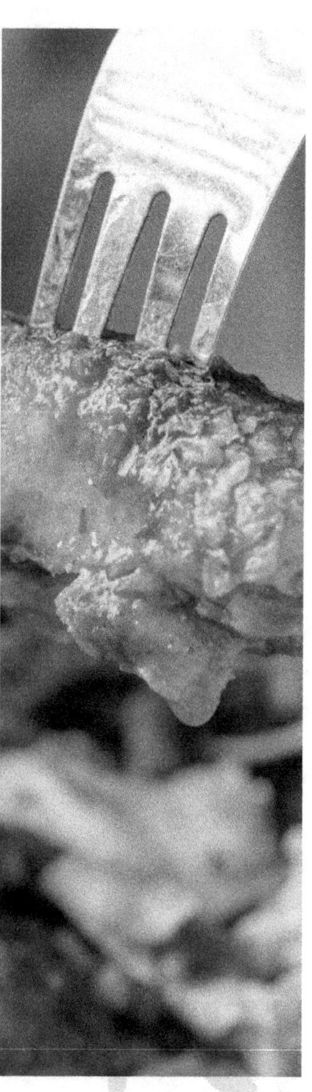

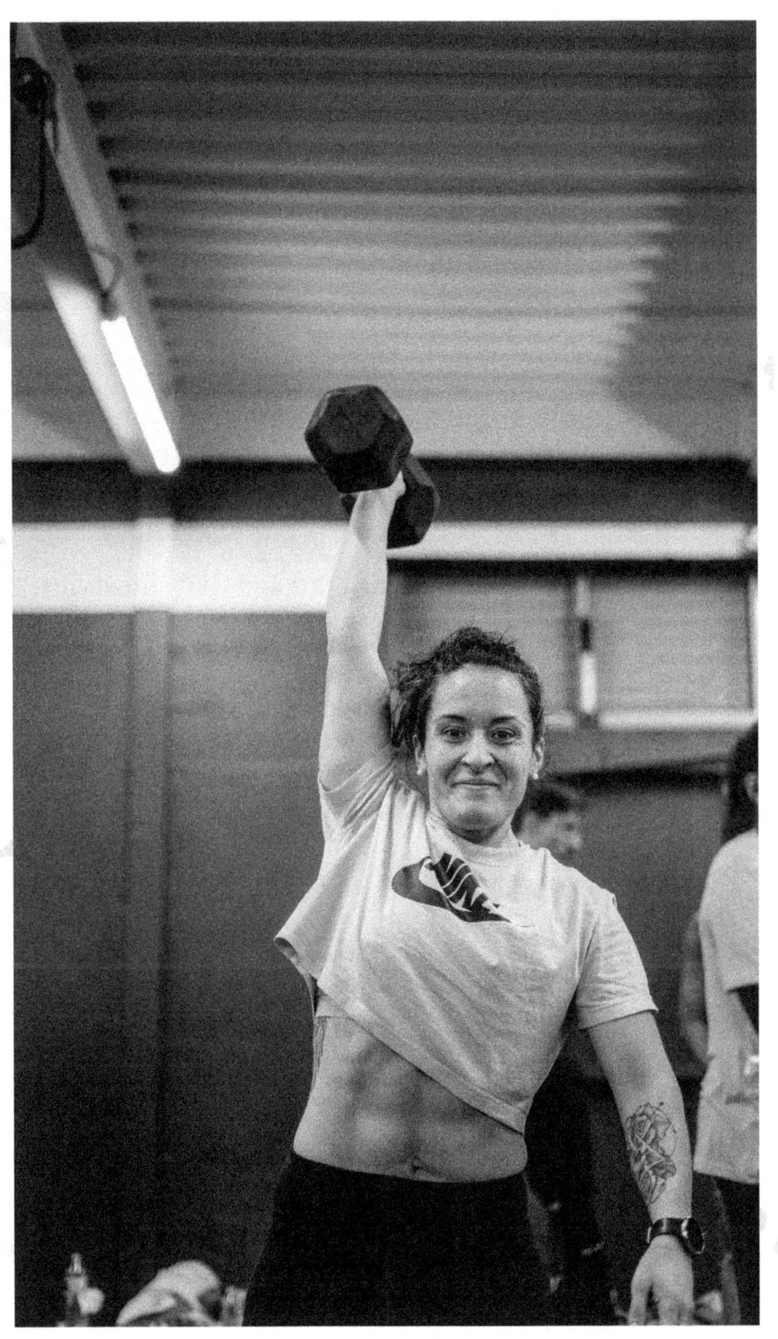

EXERCISE FOR PEOPLE WITH RESTRICTIVE LIFESTYLE

Exercise Programs for Restrictive Lifestyles

Fitting in exercise can be tough, especially with a busy or demanding lifestyle. But little adjustments may have a major impact! Here are some exercise programs tailored for people with restrictive lifestyles, proving that getting your heart rate up doesn't require a gym membership or hours of free time.

The Time-Crunched

Minute Mobs

Break up your day with quick bursts of activity. Do 10 jumping jacks, squats, or lunges every hour while at work or home.

Stair Power

Ditch the elevator and take the stairs whenever possible. This simple switch adds up throughout the day.

Commercial Cardio

Turn TV breaks into mini-workouts. Do high knees, arm circles, or stretches during commercial breaks.

The Desk Dweller

Chair Yoga

Several yoga poses can be done right from your office chair. Look for stretches for your neck, shoulders, back, and legs.

Desk De-stress

Combat sitting fatigue with quick stress-relieving exercises like neck rolls, shoulder shrugs, and deep breathing.

Walking Meetings

Ditch the conference room and have walking meetings instead. Get some steps done while keeping up with coworkers.

The Travel Warrior

Hotel Workout

Utilize hotel amenities like stairs, pools, or fitness centers for a quick workout even on the go.

In-Room Routine

No gym? No problem! Body weight exercises like lunges, planks, and push-ups can be done anywhere.

Explore on Foot

Walk or bike to explore new cities instead of relying on taxis or public transportation.

The Homebody

Household Hustle

Turn everyday chores into exercise. Vacuum with lunges, clean windows with squats, and garden with stretches.

Dance Party of One

Crank up your favorite tunes and let loose! Getting your heart rate up may be enjoyable and beneficial when you dance.

Online Workouts

Take advantage of the plethora of free workout videos online. Find routines that fit your interests and time constraints.

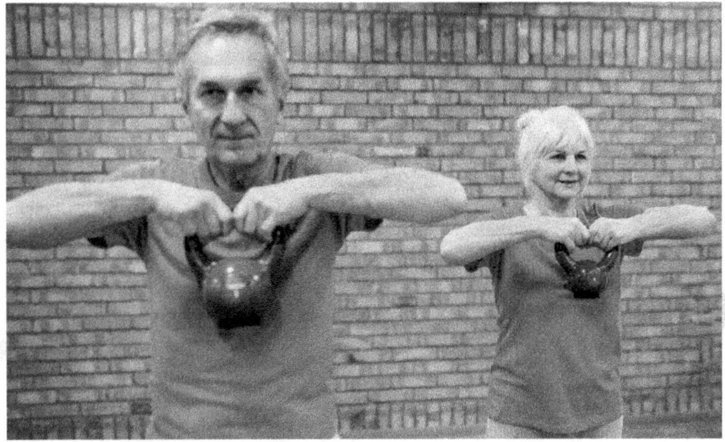

Remember:

- *Start small and gradually increase intensity and duration.*
- *Find activities you enjoy to make exercise a sustainable habit.*
- *Pay attention to your body and avoid overexerting yourself.*
- *Every little bit counts! Even short bursts of activity throughout the day make a difference.*

Tip: *Make exercise social! Find a workout buddy or join a group fitness class for added motivation and fun.*

By choosing an exercise program that fits your lifestyle and preferences, you can overcome any restrictions and start reaping the benefits of a more active life. So, lace up your shoes, put on your dancing shoes, or simply take a walk – every step counts in your journey to a healthier you!

EXERCISE FOR PEOPLE WITH SEDENTARY TO MODERATE ACTIVE LIFESTYLE

Transitioning from a sedentary life to a more active one can be daunting, but it's also incredibly rewarding! This guide offers exercise programs tailored to both ends of the spectrum, helping you find the perfect fit for your current activity level and gradually build a sustainable fitness routine.

Couch Potato to Mover

Baby Steps

Start with gentle activities like walking, swimming, or cycling for 10-15 minutes a day.

Break Up the Sitting

Set a timer for every 30 minutes and get up to stretch, walk around, or do some light housework.

Household Activities

Turn daily chores into mini-workouts. Vacuum with lunges, dust with squats, and garden with stretches.

Moderately Active to Fitness Enthusiast

Mix it Up

Combine aerobic activities like swimming, running, or dancing with strength training exercises like squats, lunges, and push-ups.

Interval Training

Alternate between periods of high-intensity activity (sprints, jumping jacks) and recovery periods (walking, jogging).

Challenge Yourself

Gradually increase the duration, intensity, and frequency of your workouts as you get fitter.

Pro-Tips for Both Levels

- **Pay attention to your body:** Avoid overexerting yourself, particularly in the beginning. Take rest days and stop if you experience pain.
- **Find activities you enjoy:** Make exercise fun by choosing activities you actually like, whether it's dancing, playing sports, or exploring nature.
- **Set realistic goals:** Start with small, achievable goals and gradually build your way up. Honoring your accomplishments along the path can help you stay inspired.
- **Embrace the outdoors:** Taking your workouts outside can boost your mood and vitamin D levels.

Exercise for People with Active and Able Lifestyle

Congratulations! Leading an active and able lifestyle is a fantastic foundation for good health and well-being. But even the most enthusiastic movers can benefit from a targeted exercise program to push their limits, prevent plateaus, and discover new ways to move their bodies. Here are some ideas to inspire your next fitness chapter:

Embrace the Power of HIIT

High-Intensity Interval Training (HIIT) is a time-efficient way to maximize your workout. Alternate between short bursts of intense activity (sprints, burpees, jumping jacks) and periods of recovery (walking, jogging). HIIT burns serious calories, boosts metabolism, and improves cardiovascular health.

Strength Train for Power and Performance

Strength training isn't just for building muscle; it improves bone density, boosts metabolism, and enhances athletic performance. Incorporate exercises that target all major muscle groups, like squats, lunges, push-ups, rows, and dead lifts. You can use body weight, free weights, resistance bands, or exercise machines.

Explore the World of Cross-Training

Break out of your routine and keep your body challenged with cross-training. This involves incorporating a variety of activities into your workout plan, such as swimming, cycling, rock climbing, dancing, or martial arts. Cross-training reduces the risk of overuse injuries, keeps things fresh and exciting, and helps you discover hidden talents.

Take Your Workouts Outdoors

Nature is a powerful motivator and a natural stress reliever. Take your workouts outside for a breath of fresh air and a change of scenery. Go for a hike, run on a trail, bike through the park, or do yoga in your backyard. Outdoor workouts can boost your mood, improve cognitive function, and strengthen your immune system.

Fuel Your Fitness with Proper Nutrition

Remember, your body is a performance machine, and it needs the right fuel to function at its best. Focus on eating a balanced diet rich in fruits, vegetables, whole grains, and lean protein. Don't forget to stay hydrated before, during, and after your workouts.

Exercise is vital, but so is recuperation and rest. Give your body time to repair and rebuild after intense workouts. Schedule rest days, get enough sleep, and practice active recovery techniques like stretching, yoga, or foam rolling.

Find Your Tribe and Make it Fun

Exercise doesn't have to be a solitary activity. Find a workout buddy or join a group fitness class to add a social element to your routine. Having someone to train with can boost your motivation, make workouts more enjoyable, and keep you accountable.

Track your workouts and progress using a fitness app or journal. This can help you stay motivated, identify areas for improvement, and celebrate your achievements.

Remember, the best exercise program is the one you'll stick with. Experiment with different activities, find what you enjoy, and make it a part of your lifestyle. With dedication and a little creativity, you can keep your fitness journey exciting and rewarding, reaching new levels of health and performance.

I hope these ideas inspire you to take your active lifestyle to the next level!

4 WEEKS EXERCISE CHALLENGE

Sedentary to Mover

Weeks	Exercise Challenge
Week 1	3x 10-15 minutes of walking
Week 2	3x 15-20 minutes of walking, adding in stretches after each session
Week 3	2x 15-20 minutes of walking, 1x 15-20 minutes of swimming or cycling
Week 4	2x 20-25 minutes of walking, 2x 15-20 minutes of body weight exercises (squats, lunges, push-ups)

Moderately Active to Fitness Enthusiast

Weeks	Exercise Challenge
Week 1	3x 30-40 minutes of cardio (running, cycling, swimming), 2x 20-30 minutes of strength training
Week 2	3x 30-40 minutes of cardio, 2x 25-35 minutes of strength training, adding interval training to 1 cardio session
Week 3	4x 30-45 minutes of cardio, 3x 25-35 minutes of strength training, incorporating different muscle groups each day
Week 4	4x 35-45 minutes of cardio, 3x 30-40 minutes of strength training, increasing intensity or duration of 1 workout each week

Remember, consistency is key! Find an exercise routine that fits your lifestyle and schedule, and stick with it. It will benefit your health and mind, I promise!

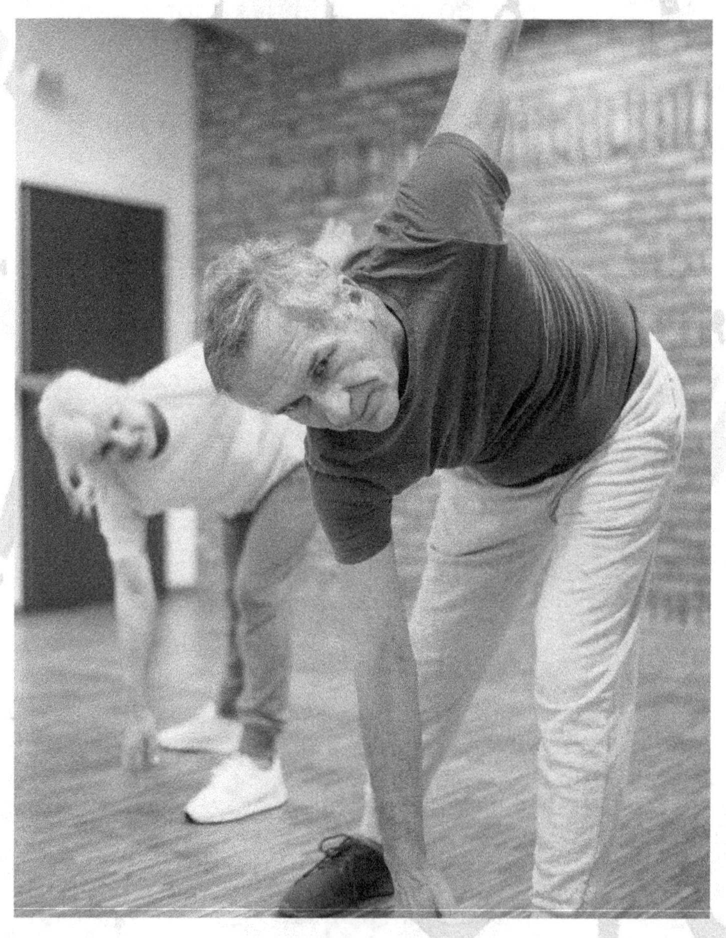

Conclusion

When you enter your 60s, your physical potential doesn't stop; rather, it begins a new chapter. This book has covered a lot of ground, including the amazing adaptability of humans, the science of strength and speed training, and the life-altering effects of taking charge of one's aging process. The people we've met are an inspiration; they've broken down barriers and given new meaning to the phrase "over the hill." Their experiences are relatable because they are examples of the ideas discussed here, not exceptions.

The main points are more than just empty clichés. Here are some measures you can take:

- Activate your body in a smart way. Try these exercises that will test your muscles, help you maintain your balance, and get your heart rate up. Pay attention to your physical limits, but don't use them as an excuse. Strength training isn't reserved for the young; it's the fountain of youth itself.

- Put gas in your tank to make it go further. Nourish your body with bright meals that encourage development and repair. Ditch the ageist myth of decline and embrace the wealth of vitality waiting to be awakened via mindful eating.
- Sharpen your mental edge. Physical fitness is interwoven with mental resilience. Embrace mindfulness, fight negativity, and approach your trip with a development mentality. You are the architect of your experience, and your viewpoint molds your reality.
- Celebrate minor successes. Don't wait for a finish line to feel successful. Every rep, every stride, every attentive breath is a win. Acknowledge your progress, celebrate milestones, and allow the pleasure of movement drive your path.

This book is not simply a tutorial; it's an invitation to a lively community. Connect with people who share your passion for surpassing expectations. Share your problems and accomplishments, take inspiration in other experiences, and become a light of encouragement yourself. Remember, age is only a number. The potential for power, speed, and vitality lies inside everyone of us, regardless of the wrinkles on our faces or the grey in our hair.

So, my reader, what are you waiting for? The world is your gym, your kitchen is your laboratory, and your intellect is the most powerful instrument at your disposal. Take the initial step, accept the ideas you've learnt, and go on your own incredible adventure of strength and speed. It's never too late to alter the story of aging. Go out, defy expectations, and become the fittest, quickest, and most vivacious version of yourself, year after year, decade after decade. The world awaits your victory lap.

Now, get out there and show them what "60 and beyond" actually means!

Frequent Asks Questions

When Can I Start Lifting Weights?

AGE IS ONLY A NUMBER!

EVERYONE'S AGE IS RELATIVE.

THERE IS ALWAYS MORE TO COME!

There are seniors all throughout the globe proving that you can accomplish everything you set your mind to, regardless of your age!

Irene O'Shea, became the oldest skydiver in the world when she was 102 years old.

Even at the age of 104, Fauja Singh was still going strong, finishing marathons.

Gymnast Johanna Quaas competed at the age of 92.

Ernestine Shepherd, who is 83 years old and still bodybuilding, is a personal trainer.

No kind of strength training is inappropriate for someone of your age.

I have helped hundreds of individuals increase their strength and grow muscle from the ages of 54 (or younger), all the way up to 104. 104 and flourishing!

You are also not too old to accomplish whatever else you wish to do.

So, if you hold the idea that age is a reason not to undertake anything. Then chuck it out!

If someone attempts to destroy your goals with the "you're too old" excuse, toss them out too!

'Age' is never a cause to not accomplish anything. Especially weights!

anything age you are, do anything you want to do, and have fun doing it!

Won't I injure Myself If I Lift Weights?

If you experience this concern, you are not alone!

This is a frequent anxiety encountered by individuals new to strength training, particularly when it comes to lifting weights.

YES!..... There IS a possibility you could hurt or harm yourself undertaking strength workouts!

And, our odds of harming oneself DOES rise as we become older, and we DO increase our risk by exercising with weights.

However.... This concern is unjustified!

"I've had a lot of worries in my life, most of which never happened."

— Mark Twain

The advantages of strength training significantly exceed the slight danger of harming oneself.

I can guarantee you, If you conduct strength training appropriately (as explained in this article), strength training is entirely safe and the odds of you harming yourself are close to zilch!

As you continue strength training, with your now stronger, steadier physique, you'll have far less risk of harming yourself in general.

You'll also realize that strength training wasn't something to dread and it becomes easy and fun once you get the hang of it.

Ok! Some of you may never find strength training entertaining, however, you'll see and feel the advantages eventually and want to to keep it up!

Based on your existing skills, strength levels or health state, you may need to alter the exercises or your program in some manner so that you can complete them safely. (This, and more will be explored inside this text).

But good strength training is great for everyone, and safe, no matter your age!

You're just as competent as everyone else!

Exercise Log Book

EXERCISE LOG BOOK/TRACKER

DATE: / /

MORNING ROUTINE M T W T F S S

HEALTH + WELLNESS M T W T F S S

SELF-CARE + WELLBEING M T W T F S S

EVENING ROUTINE M T W T F S S

EXERCISE LOG BOOK/TRACKER

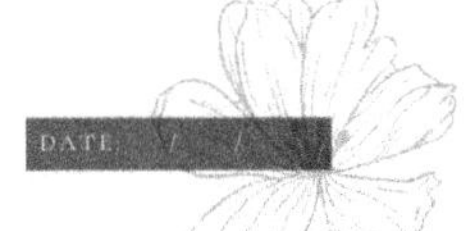

MORNING ROUTINE	M	T	W	T	F	S	S
	○	○	○	○	○	○	○
	○	○	○	○	○	○	○
	○	○	○	○	○	○	○
	○	○	○	○	○	○	○
	○	○	○	○	○	○	○

HEALTH + WELLNESS	M	T	W	T	F	S	S
	○	○	○	○	○	○	○
	○	○	○	○	○	○	○
	○	○	○	○	○	○	○
	○	○	○	○	○	○	○
	○	○	○	○	○	○	○

SELF-CARE + WELLBEING	M	T	W	T	F	S	S
	○	○	○	○	○	○	○
	○	○	○	○	○	○	○
	○	○	○	○	○	○	○
	○	○	○	○	○	○	○
	○	○	○	○	○	○	○

EVENING ROUTINE	M	T	W	T	F	S	S
	○	○	○	○	○	○	○
	○	○	○	○	○	○	○
	○	○	○	○	○	○	○
	○	○	○	○	○	○	○
	○	○	○	○	○	○	○

EXERCISE LOG BOOK/TRACKER

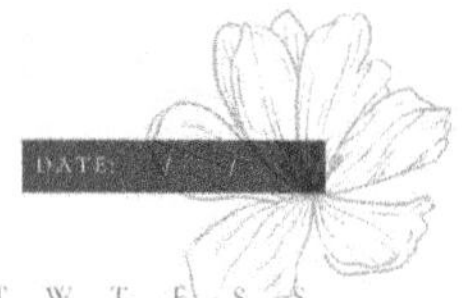

MORNING ROUTINE	M	T	W	T	F	S	S
	○	○	○	○	○	○	○
	○	○	○	○	○	○	○
	○	○	○	○	○	○	○
	○	○	○	○	○	○	○
	○	○	○	○	○	○	○

HEALTH + WELLNESS	M	T	W	T	F	S	S
	○	○	○	○	○	○	○
	○	○	○	○	○	○	○
	○	○	○	○	○	○	○
	○	○	○	○	○	○	○
	○	○	○	○	○	○	○

SELF-CARE + WELLBEING	M	T	W	T	F	S	S
	○	○	○	○	○	○	○
	○	○	○	○	○	○	○
	○	○	○	○	○	○	○
	○	○	○	○	○	○	○
	○	○	○	○	○	○	○

EVENING ROUTINE	M	T	W	T	F	S	S
	○	○	○	○	○	○	○
	○	○	○	○	○	○	○
	○	○	○	○	○	○	○
	○	○	○	○	○	○	○
	○	○	○	○	○	○	○

EXERCISE LOG BOOK/TRACKER

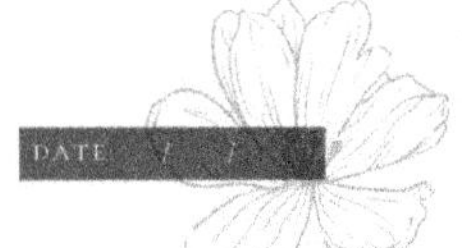

MORNING ROUTINE	M	T	W	T	F	S	S
	○	○	○	○	○	○	○
	○	○	○	○	○	○	○
	○	○	○	○	○	○	○
	○	○	○	○	○	○	○
	○	○	○	○	○	○	○

HEALTH + WELLNESS	M	T	W	T	F	S	S
	○	○	○	○	○	○	○
	○	○	○	○	○	○	○
	○	○	○	○	○	○	○
	○	○	○	○	○	○	○
	○	○	○	○	○	○	○

SELF-CARE + WELLBEING	M	T	W	T	F	S	S
	○	○	○	○	○	○	○
	○	○	○	○	○	○	○
	○	○	○	○	○	○	○
	○	○	○	○	○	○	○
	○	○	○	○	○	○	○

EVENING ROUTINE	M	T	W	T	F	S	S
	○	○	○	○	○	○	○
	○	○	○	○	○	○	○
	○	○	○	○	○	○	○
	○	○	○	○	○	○	○
	○	○	○	○	○	○	○

EXERCISE LOG BOOK/TRACKER

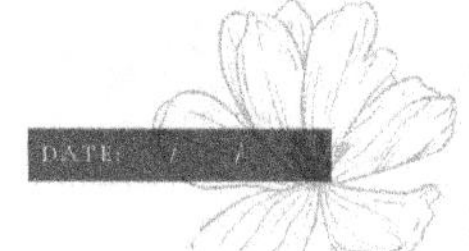

MORNING ROUTINE

M T W T F S S

HEALTH + WELLNESS

M T W T F S S

SELF-CARE + WELLBEING

M T W T F S S

EVENING ROUTINE

M T W T F S S

EXERCISE LOG BOOK/TRACKER

MORNING ROUTINE	M	T	W	T	F	S	S
	○	○	○	○	○	○	○
	○	○	○	○	○	○	○
	○	○	○	○	○	○	○
	○	○	○	○	○	○	○
	○	○	○	○	○	○	○

HEALTH + WELLNESS	M	T	W	T	F	S	S
	○	○	○	○	○	○	○
	○	○	○	○	○	○	○
	○	○	○	○	○	○	○
	○	○	○	○	○	○	○
	○	○	○	○	○	○	○

SELF-CARE + WELLBEING	M	T	W	T	F	S	S
	○	○	○	○	○	○	○
	○	○	○	○	○	○	○
	○	○	○	○	○	○	○
	○	○	○	○	○	○	○
	○	○	○	○	○	○	○

EVENING ROUTINE	M	T	W	T	F	S	S
	○	○	○	○	○	○	○
	○	○	○	○	○	○	○
	○	○	○	○	○	○	○
	○	○	○	○	○	○	○
	○	○	○	○	○	○	○

EXERCISE LOG BOOK/TRACKER

MORNING ROUTINE	M	T	W	T	F	S	S
	○	○	○	○	○	○	○
	○	○	○	○	○	○	○
	○	○	○	○	○	○	○
	○	○	○	○	○	○	○
	○	○	○	○	○	○	○

HEALTH + WELLNESS	M	T	W	T	F	S	S
	○	○	○	○	○	○	○
	○	○	○	○	○	○	○
	○	○	○	○	○	○	○
	○	○	○	○	○	○	○
	○	○	○	○	○	○	○

SELF-CARE + WELLBEING	M	T	W	T	F	S	S
	○	○	○	○	○	○	○
	○	○	○	○	○	○	○
	○	○	○	○	○	○	○
	○	○	○	○	○	○	○
	○	○	○	○	○	○	○

EVENING ROUTINE	M	T	W	T	F	S	S
	○	○	○	○	○	○	○
	○	○	○	○	○	○	○
	○	○	○	○	○	○	○
	○	○	○	○	○	○	○
	○	○	○	○	○	○	○

Printed in the USA
CPSIA information can be obtained
at www.ICGtesting.com
LVHW010330100624
782791LV00009B/899

9 798878 205184